10 REASONS DOGS ARE THE ABSOLUTE BEST:

A BOOK OF TINY TAILS

Amanda Gist

Illustrations by

Douglas Gist

Soulful Creative Studios
PO Box 18443
Reno, NV 89511

Ordering Information:
Quantity sales. Special discounts are available on quantity purchases by corporations, associations, and others. For details, contact the "Special Sales Department" at the address above.

10 Reasons Dogs Are the Absolute Best: A Book of Tiny Tails/ Amanda Gist. —1st ed.
ISBN 978-1-7353711-0-8

"We give dogs time we can spare, space we can spare, and love we can spare. And in return, dogs give us their all. It's the best deal man has ever made." M. Facklam

10 Reasons Dogs Are the Absolute Best

Table of Contents

Dedicated to Haylie Denae, a lifetime wouldn't be long enough.

10 Reasons Dogs Are the Absolute Best

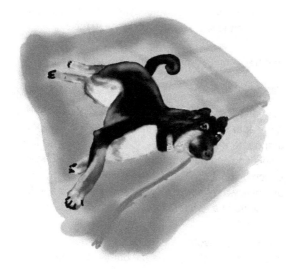

She was the quietest one out of all of them. The perfect size for me, around 35 pounds and "full grown," they told me. A year old. She had beautiful markings and beautiful eyes and a sweet face and a tail that curled up like a pig's and she was looking at me with this look that told me all she wanted was a one-way ticket out of there and maybe a few French fries.

But I was still unsure. This would be so much responsibility for such a not responsible person. My food usually went bad in the fridge, how would I keep a dog alive? A living, breathing thing that needed me to care for them as a means of their survival? God that sounded scary. But I wanted a dog so badly. I had just gone through a horrendous breakup and needed something in my corner. Something to love me. Something I could love. I had grown up with dogs since the day I was born and knew loving was their main skill and something they were phenomenal at, but I was still afraid she would go the way of the food in the fridge.

So I left her.

The next day was Thanksgiving, 2007. It feels like a lifetime ago and also just yesterday as I write this, her soft snore filling my apartment. I spent Thanksgiving with my family at my grandparent's home that year, and even with all the incredible cooking and stories being told and wine spills on the couch, I spent my Thanksgiving with her on my mind. All I could think was, *I don't want her to ever spend another holiday alone in a kennel again.*

And so Friday, November 23rd, 2007, the day after Thanksgiving, we officially began our lives together.

I had no idea what I was doing. I was still crossing my fingers this dog wouldn't end up like the food in the fridge. I hadn't even really tried plants yet, I had just made the leap straight from trying to keep veggies fresh to trying to keep a dog alive. However, I was unaware that I was embarking on what would be one of many challenges with her and that perhaps, in hindsight, I might have bought myself a nice bamboo plant instead.

Thank God I didn't.

40 pounds (yes, "full grown," they said…) and about a year of disciplining and training and losing my mind later, I finally had a dog I could handle on my hands. Her name: Haylie Denae. Her love language: French fries (I had gotten this right on the first day). Her zodiac sign: Gemini (I had decided, having doubled in size, she was closer to only six months old when I adopted her and hence, was born in May). Her most amazing discovery: snow. Her favorite toy: my underwear hot out of the dryer. Go figure.

13 years have passed now and I write this book in honor of Haylie Denae and the stories we've accumulated together. I write it as a thank you for that time she saved my life (we'll get to that). I write it to share the ways she's made my life better, and to remind you of the ways your dog has made your life better. I write it for everyone who has ever had a dog turn out to be *the* best thing that ever happened to them. And I write it for those of us who are holding on tight, knowing in the back of our minds, some of us in the forefront, that eventually the day is coming, and not knowing how we will get through it. This book is to serve as your reminder of the gifts your dog has given you. The ones you'll carry in your heart forever, right next to their paw print.

10 Reasons Dogs Are the Absolute Best

"To err is human - to forgive, canine."
Author Unknown

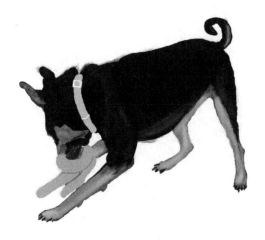

10 Reasons Dogs Are the Absolute Best

had only been renting this beautiful home for a few months. It was two stories, had a single car garage, a his-and-hers master bathroom, and huge eastern-facing bedroom windows that let all the light in as the sun came up - my favorite part. And here I was, sitting against the living room wall of my beautiful home, sobbing, while a trail of coffee grounds and kitchen trash lead to a huge puddle of red Kool-aid soaking into the carpet. Haylie was running circles around the coffee table at the speed of light, tracking the Kool-aid into a kaleidoscope pattern throughout the carpet with her paws.

I had already tried the stern voice, which turned into the yelling at her as my adult-sized frustration grew into Hulk-sized frustration. I had tried grabbing at her, but she was apparently by some freak accident bred with cheetah and too fast to catch. I had even tried the thing you're not supposed to try when the puppy is acting out - *treats.* I knew I wasn't supposed to reward her for her behavior, but I was desperate to get her attention long enough to grab her collar and grasp some semblance of control over the situation. Nothing worked.

This was the first of many times I got the idea in my head to take Haylie back to where I got her and surrender her. This thought compounded the heightened emotions I was already experiencing and added this onslaught of heavy guilt to the mix; I was already attached to this little girl, and yet here I was, thinking about taking her back. Because I couldn't handle her. Because she was completely out of control. Because I had no idea what to do. Because she was nothing like the sweet, quiet girl I met at the kennel. Because they had lied to me.

She wasn't a year old; she was maybe six months. She wasn't a shepherd mix; I learned later she had a breed called Basenji in her, a breed that is recommended to be bought or adopted in pairs so they can wear each other out because they have so much unrelenting energy to burn.

These weren't even the type of behavioral issues obedience training dealt with. She could sit and stay like a champ *when she wanted to* and had a graduation certificate to prove it. She was smarter than the average bear. And too smart for her own good. And mine.

I had no idea where to turn, what to do, or who to go to for help. And at the moment I was so exhausted I couldn't even fathom getting through this with her.

So there I sat. Crying like a loon, yelling at Haylie each time she rounded the corner of the coffee table racetrack, frustrated, angry, guilty, sad, all of the emotions. A real winner. And then, as she began to tire herself out and I began to totally give up, she walked right up to me with her little pig tail curled up in the air and her ears back and licked the snot and tears off my face.

She still just wanted to love me.

Through the anger, the frustration, the tears, the guilt, she just wanted to love me. At one of my worst moments. The moment I was thinking about giving her back. She just wanted to love me. *Me.* If she had been a person and had known I was thinking about giving her back, she wouldn't have wanted anything to do with me. But this is the magic in dogs. *They just want to love us.* Regardless of which version of *us* we're displaying.

They want to love the us that's angry with them for chewing a hole in our favorite hoodie. They want to love the us that just lost our job. They want to love the us that got broken up with and can't breathe through the sobs. They want to love the us that has food in our hand *and* the us that doesn't.

They want to love the us that makes bad decisions sometimes, hurts others sometimes, doesn't always say the right thing, and has bad habits. The us we can't always show other people. They want to love *that* us.

And for some of us, they're the only ones that do.

10 Reasons Dogs Are the Absolute Best

CH. 2 They surprise you in the best of ways

"Buy a pup and your money will buy love unflinching." R. Kipling

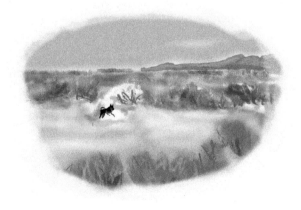

10 Reasons Dogs Are the Absolute Best

"**H**aylie!" My family and I called out, over and over. I was sick to my stomach, my heart felt like it would beat right out of my chest. I don't think I'd ever felt fear in my life like I did that night. What if she was actually gone? What if I'd lost her? What if I had to live with having lost her for the rest of my life? What if something awful happened to her? What if I was leaving her in a field just like she was found in a field when she was turned in to the rescue shelter? The *what ifs* were drowning me as I kept searching for her black body to appear in the white snow.

I had a large pond behind my new apartment (I moved a lot) surrounded by land that wasn't built up yet, just dirt and brush. There was a beautiful paved walking path all the way around it and I'd begun taking Haylie halfway around the lake and then releasing her from her leash and letting her run to burn some of her energy off. We'd been having much calmer nights once this became part of our routine, but tonight she'd disappeared behind a small hill and as I went towards where she had been, she was no longer in sight. I began panicking and calling her name, but her little face never came bouncing back toward me like it always had, her paws throwing snow to the sides like an Alaskan sled dog in a race.

I called and called for her through the tears and snot rolling down my flushed face. I couldn't go back home without her. I wouldn't. It was around four in the afternoon and I was desperate to find her before dark.

I called my dad in that state of panic that daughters call their dads in that makes the dads wonder if their daughters still have all their limbs. Through the crying I could barely get out the words to share the story, but he and my mom quickly drove the two freeway exits down they lived from my new home and we combined efforts searching.

21

We searched and searched, the visceral pain in my heart growing and expanding as the minutes wore on. Dusk started to fall early, as it always does in winter. Soon dark began to follow. The street lights flickered on, the traffic began to increase as we closed in on five o'clock, then six o'clock, and commuters began rushing home.

My parents didn't tell me we were going home for the night, they told me we were going home to "regroup." Warm up. Game plan. But I was devastated. I couldn't imagine walking through my front door and leaving her out in the dark and cold, God only knew where, and in what kind of danger. But I was also exhausted, and maybe I *needed* to regroup. I didn't know what I needed at that point. I just knew I needed to go back to the second I took her off that leash and undo all of it, take it back, rewind it, have her safely six feet in front of me clipped into her black nylon harness on her black nylon leash looking back at me.

My dad's truck slowly pulled into my apartment's driveway and crept through the parking lot toward my building. I don't remember if I was crying still but I can't imagine I had any tears left at that point. He parked in a guest spot and we all shuffled out and crossed the slushy pavement toward my unit, no one saying a word, a collective silent agreement to not talk about the thing that must eventually be talked about.

I walked toward my bottom floor apartment with an empty heart and hollow feeling in my stomach, knowing I'd have to open that front door without her wiggling butt running up to greet me. As I got closer to my front patio, I broke down in tears, kind of like I'm breaking down in tears right now just remembering the emotionally-charged moment. There she stood; standing tall, waiting for me on the patio like nothing had happened and I should've known I'd find her there.

You should know, at this point, my laptop screen is blurry through the eyeball wetness as I type this. I got to the patio and got down on my knees and wept into her fur, while she stood there confused and wondering why I was so dramatic. We all went inside and the weeping turned into alternating bouts of weeping and laughing at the irony, then back to weeping with pure relief.

I hadn't had a cell in my body confident that she knew her way home. We hadn't lived in that apartment for long. But that night I learned I had to give her much more credit. She not only knew her way home, she knew that seeing her standing there would be one of the most cherished surprises of my life. And to this day, it still is.

10 Reasons Dogs Are the Absolute Best

"Dogs have boundless enthusiasm but no sense of shame. I should have a dog as a life coach."
Moby

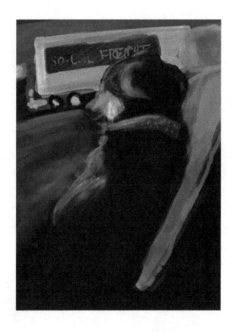

10 Reasons Dogs Are the Absolute Best

'd gotten a job through an old co-worker. I didn't know much about it, but it seemed promising. Something about doing assistant work for a couple that owned a clothing line. I could do it. I could definitely do it if it got me out of my hometown, where I was still reeling from an awful breakup eight months earlier and everywhere I went reminded me of him.

My relationship had ended. My lease was ending. The nightclub I worked at was closing. I had nothing keeping me there. So I took the job.

It was a whirlwind week of telling my parents I was moving to Los Angeles, packing as much as I could fit into my little Mustang, and making plans for somehow making this work as an irresponsible 22-year-old who had zero life experience and big dreams of a life beyond where she grew up.

I had to leave Haylie with my parents for three weeks, the longest I'd ever been away from her, the longest I've been away from her to this day. But I was going to be hotel hopping until I found a place to live and trying to set up a life for us, and my mom and dad had talked me into the fact that taking her with me would make things infinitely harder for myself. I had to drive back up for a surprise birthday party in three weeks, so I would take her down to LA with me then.

It was possibly the loneliest three weeks of my life. No one to talk to while I ate my continental breakfast in my hotel rooms. No one to visit me in the bathroom for back scratches while I peed. No one to cuddle with me in bed at night like Haylie loved to do before settling down at the foot of the bed where she could protect me from monsters and burglars at first sight. The only blessing is that those three weeks are mostly a blur of hotel rooms and apartment tours

27

and getting cut off in traffic, being a kind driver in a quite unkind driving environment.

Eventually I settled on a studio apartment overlooking city lights in a building that bumped up to the beach on the opposite side. One that I didn't even really know if I could afford on my meager assistant monthly salary but one where there weren't people sleeping in the front doorway or fires in the dumpster, although I ended up putting in my time living in one of those neighborhoods also.

At the end of the three weeks I was *so* eager to get back home to Haylie. My heart had been walking around outside of my chest and 500 miles away for too long and as I pulled in the driveway I could just imagine the smell of the excitement and urination on the floor as she jumped around like an acrobat on steroids.

We reunited in the laundry room at my parents' house and there was pee and tears and big smiles from both of us and lots of kisses. I'm convinced she thought I was never coming back for her. I even mailed her a card while I was gone for Mom to read to her letting her know I was, in fact, coming back. I hated the thought of her even feeling the least bit abandoned by me.

A few days later, I packed the Mustang full again with the rest of what I could fit into it while allowing special space for a special dog in the front seat. We said our goodbyes and this time we both piled into the leather bucket seats and pulled out of the driveway to embark on the adventure of a lifetime.

Haylie was the ultimate road trip buddy. Not once did she change the radio, ask to stop for a potty break, or talk too much. She slept. She looked out the window at the huge 18-wheelers accompanying us on our drive south. She looked over at me, making sure I was still in this with her. She peed like a champ when asked to, ate snacks when offered to her, and enjoyed the windows open. Also, she was cute to look at, a bonus.

Eventually the sun began going down, the air became humid and thick, and we began trading brush and tall grasses for palm trees. The freeway took us through North Hollywood, then Hollywood, brightly colored lights marking famous places to eat and drink and faces like Marilyn's graffitied in black and white across concrete walls. Then we made our way through downtown LA, Haylie staring up at the cityscape of buildings taller than anything she'd ever seen. Eventually we made it to our apartment building, and after a quick pee on the front lawn, Haylie and I took an elevator up 12 flights to our studio apartment, where I introduced her to the first of many new homes we would live in over the next five years, in a city where we would laugh, cry, and grow together.

For better or worse.

10 Reasons Dogs Are the Absolute Best

"Dogs are not our whole life, but they make our lives whole." R. Caras

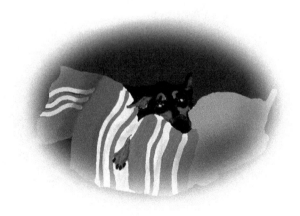

10 Reasons Dogs Are the Absolute Best

t's many years, one big move, and a mental breakdown later. I walk in the front door, the small light above the stove casting shadows around the small apartment. Haylie bounces off the bed where she was watching my car pull in through the window and makes her way to the front door to greet me. I set my big bag of tricks down, the one that holds my lunch for work and notebooks and calendars and so much more. I kick off my fancy shiny black Crocs, which are just a given if you're a healthcare worker, and sink into the leather recliner. Haylie jumps up onto my lap with her two front paws, covering my black scrubs in fur but also providing me much-needed love at the end of my always-awful days at the psychiatric hospital, so the fur is acceptable.

We sit like this for a while, her getting scratches behind the ears and me getting peace and quiet out of the deal. My day runs through my head; every patient that reminded me of myself and my depression. Every hospital chart I read that disclosed how the suicide attempt happened. Every moment I wondered if this is what my future held, a revolving door of mental hospital stays.

I had moved back to my hometown from LA after five years, struggling with severe bulimia and depression, and had finally been diagnosed as bipolar shortly after. While a psychiatric hospital was probably the last place I should've been working, I had the strongest desire to help those who had felt what I had felt, who were where I had been. The problem was, I hadn't "been" there. I *was* there. I was still in the middle of it. I wasn't well; I wasn't mentally healthy. So I still came home each night haunted by what my day entailed, with questions I didn't have answers to.

I had recently made a deal with my psychiatrist. Instead of coming home, having an anxiety attack, and spinning out mentally reliving my day at the hospital, I would create a *relaxation routine.* This relaxation routine was mine, all mine. I would curate it, I would be responsible for following through with it, and I would reap the benefits.

My relaxation routine was messy at first. I didn't exactly know *how* to relax. I had been fighting with my mental health for years now, and relaxation hadn't been part of the game plan. It took me awhile to curate my relaxation routine, but it eventually ended up looking something like this: getting into my pajamas, all the lights turned out, a few scented candles lit (usually scents like lavender and eucalyptus, calming and soothing), a fuzzy blanket over me on the couch, Haylie curled up in her bed next to the couch, and the Spring Baking Championship on tv. Now there was also Kids' Baking Championship and Holiday Baking Championship, but when I started this practice, it was Spring Baking Championship. Duff Goldman was my favorite.

Haylie snored while I watched the contestants ice cupcakes against the clock. It was then that I discovered there was something about baking and cooking shows that soothed me, and helped send Haylie off to sleep. It was only a matter of minutes before she would have her eyes closed once the tv went on. She rarely even made it to the show's opening credits and the judge introduction.

We'd exist in this space together, this relaxation routine, for 45 minutes to an hour each night, her resting and snoring in rhythm and me coming down from the day with the mesmerizing swirls of frosting and marble cookies.

Eventually I'd get up and blow out the candles, she'd lift her little head sleepily, and we'd softly cross the living room, off to bed together.

It turned out my psychiatrist knew what he was talking about. Instead of anxious and overwhelmed, I'd find myself relaxed and would drift right to sleep, Haylie curled up at my feet, exhausted from her Baking Championship-length nap. She turned out to be a key piece to my relaxation routine - her soft snores keeping time and reminding me I wasn't alone. To this day, although we've now made it through all of the Baking Championships and are currently watching Gordon in Hell's Kitchen - it's her and I in the living room, food on the tv, and candles burning to erase the day.

Who knew dog snores and television carbs would be my mental saving grace?

10 Reasons Dogs Are the Absolute Best

"A well-trained dog will make no attempt to share your lunch. He will just make you feel so guilty that you cannot enjoy it." H. Thomson

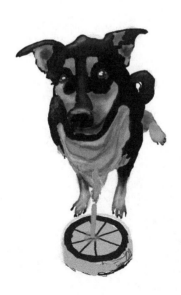

10 Reasons Dogs Are the Absolute Best

was in the kitchen in the middle of cooking frijoles fresca bowls for my parents and sister, my hair sticking to the back of my neck with sweat in my small apartment. They would be here soon, their cream and coral-colored invitations with Haylie's picture on them said six o'clock and it was about five 'til. We were having an adoptiversary party for Haylie and I, as it was a few days after our 12 year anniversary and she had just been diagnosed with B-cell lymphoma a couple of months before. I didn't know how long she would be here and I wanted to celebrate her.

I carefully set out a made-for-dogs celebration pie, some chocolate cupcakes, chips and salsa, a veggie tray with tomatoes, carrots, celery, and ranch dressing, cute little wine glasses, and a couple bottles. There were paper plates with Haylie's face on them that said *Happy 12th Adoptiversary!* There were napkins with Haylie's face on them and little succulents I'd potted as party favors with tags that had Haylie's face on them, basically Haylie was everywhere, including running around the apartment in her coral and gold handkerchief excited for whatever was about to happen.

While I was busy wondering how anyone ever in the history of man hosted Thanksgiving because I was stressed to the max hosting three family members, said family members showed up at my door. They came in with a bustle of excitement and hello's to Haylie and I, a party bag on my mom's arm and smiles on their faces. Haylie ran to greet them and show off her handkerchief right before she dunked it in water trying to get a drink and proceeded to fling water all over the floors. She's not the most graceful, but she tries.

Everyone settled down into their seats and I kept whirling around the kitchen, putting the finishing touches on dinner. Haylie enjoyed some hand-fed tortilla chips and bounced around the apartment, clearly feeling so much better from the two months of chemo she'd undergone at that point than she had felt when she was diagnosed, weak and barely eating. It was amazing to see her this way, she was engaged and interactive and enjoying having company, even if she had no idea what we were celebrating or that they were there for her.

Tortilla chips had always been one of her favorites, right up there with French fries. We had an arrangement: when I brought home Mexican takeout like Chipotle or Q'Doba, I'd share my tortilla chips with her. When I brought home any other takeout, I'd share my French fries with her. She always got something out of the deal. When she was a puppy this was a given because she would steal, and I still to this day believe she stole with no regrets or guilt. As she got older, sharing with her became a given because I couldn't *not* share with her as she patiently watched me eat with her big brown eyes and floppy ears perked up, just silently reminding me she was there and "hungry." Always hungry. Always, always hungry.

As I had my back turned at the stove, among all the tortilla chips, mom decided to try a carrot. Apparently Haylie not only took it, but loved it and looked back up for more as soon as she finished it. This is how we learned that carrots were also a favorite. She now gets her own one pound bag of carrots every week on our grocery shopping trip.

Her other favorites?

- Graham crackers
- Cottage cheese
- String cheese
- Ground turkey*
- Scrambled eggs*

- Sushi (yes, sushi)
- Tortillas

...this is not a comprehensive list, but all I can think of at the moment.

*This was her chemo diet when she wouldn't eat dog food. Scrambled eggs in the morning and ground turkey at night. Fun fact: I cooked more for her during that time than I did for myself.

10 Reasons Dogs Are the Absolute Best

CH. 6 They comfort you in your absolute hardest moments

"I have found that when you are deeply troubled, there are things you get from the silent devoted companionship of a dog that you can get from no other source." D. Day

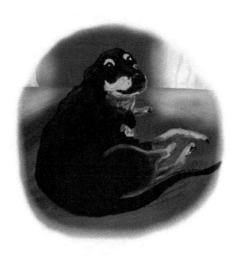

10 Reasons Dogs Are the Absolute Best

felt like I was on fire and no one could see me. No one could see my flesh burning, my soul leaving my body, smoke drifting above me, signaling distress. So instead of throwing water on me, they kept throwing medications and therapy sessions at me. Because no one had the answers. No one. So I kept burning.

She stayed by my side, every second of every day. From the moment my eyes opened in the morning, when the enormous weight of having to go through another day in this dark place, in this pain, held me down in my bed. To the evenings, climbing back into bed at four o'clock, five o'clock in the afternoon, if not earlier. Watching the shade of the paint on the walls change as the sun set outside my windows, proof that the world carried on without me.

She slept as many hours as I did, even if that meant 24 of them in a row, her body silently supportive next to me in bed. She'd raise her head every once in a while, looking back at me, looking me in the eyes. She saw the fire. And she knew all she could do to help was be present. So she did that.

Severe depression took over my life for many years in my late twenties and early thirties. At this time I didn't have a boyfriend or husband, kids. I lived alone with the exception of Haylie. I often think she's the only soul on this earth that doesn't, won't, judge me - because she's truly seen the worst minutes of time slip by that no one else has. She's experienced those worst minutes of time with me, by my side, never even going to the door to be let out or her water bowl to drink. She somehow, miraculously, spent the time I was debilitated by depression and bound to my bed by an invisible force with me, really *with me;* she met me where I was and never tried to make me be somewhere else.

She'd be at the end of the bed, and I'd wake up, move my foot so it was touching her, and fall back asleep, with a little more comfort than I had before, knowing she was there.

When I'd try to get up, to shower, to leave my house, and I couldn't, the invisible force kept me on the edge of my bed too exhausted to re-enter the world, I'd lay back down with more comfort knowing she would stay there with me as long as I needed.

When the numbness and emptiness would shift into sadness and the crying would begin, what felt like endless crying, I'd experience comfort when she'd get up and move next to me, lying down face-to-face with me, licking the salty tears from my skin.

She wasn't disappointed in me for not getting better, faster. She didn't judge me for how dysfunctional I'd become as a human being. She didn't love me any less on the 100th day in bed than she loved me on the first day in bed.

One of Haylie's superpowers is her empathy. I'll forever be indebted to her for the comfort she brought me during that time in my life, and the comfort she brings during subsequent depressive episodes year after year. No amount of graham crackers or carrots can pay her back for the consistency and support she unknowingly gave me, becoming my rock while the days and nights blurred around me.

As the bumper sticker says, *who rescued who?*

"Dogs do speak, but only to those who know how to listen." O. Pamuk

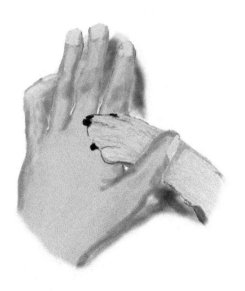

10 Reasons Dogs Are the Absolute Best

sat on the kitchen floor with my back against the cupboards. The apartment was dark, the small light above the stove casting harsh, sharp shadows off the counters and refrigerator. I leaned my head back against the cupboard door, closed my eyes, and took several deep breaths. But I felt the anxiety rushing back in, the voices talking in circles but at the same time, clearly, articulately, in my head. The impulsivity vibrating in my hands.

The green digital clock on the stove glowed 12:04 A.M. It was the middle of the night, I'd just gotten home from work about a half hour earlier. I'd been here before. Night shifts at the psychiatric hospital often ended this way that summer, summer of 2018. Some nights I never made it to my relaxation routine, because I got caught before that. I got caught before I made it into my pajamas. Before I brushed my teeth. Before I lit the candles. Before I turned Spring Baking Championship on. I got caught as soon as I walked into the kitchen to take my nighttime medications, trying to stay on some semblance of a schedule by taking them as soon as I got home from work. But some nights it was a trap. Some nights my mental state and the day I'd had and the things I'd seen and heard at the hospital and the endless bottles of medications I had on my countertop all lined up and I'd sink onto the floor, with a bottle in my hand, fighting myself.

Haylie sat in front of me in the kitchen, the features of her face shadowed and her eyes peering into mine. She never took the pill bottle out of my hand. Never called 911. Never said a word to talk me out of it. But she saved my life, over and over that summer, because I would think to myself, *she would be so confused if I was gone.* And, *no one would ever love her the way I love her.*

So I'd set the pills aside and put each hand on the sides of her face and let her lick the tears from my cheeks while I cried, partly out of relief that the impulse to take my life was slowly passing and partly out of the pain of experiencing this nightmare of a night again and again.

Without knowing it, she kept me here. All because she just knew when I needed her. She knew when to meet me on the kitchen floor instead of stay curled up in her bed. She knew when to protect me from myself.

She knew to take the pill bottle out of my hand in the only way she knew how.

"Fall in love with a dog, and in many ways you enter a new orbit, a universe that features not just new colors but new rituals, new rules, a new way of experiencing attachment." C. Knapp

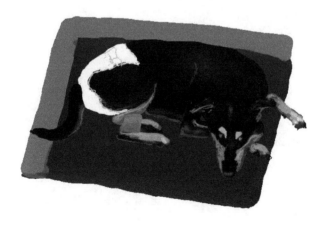

10 Reasons Dogs Are the Absolute Best

I woke up that morning and crawled down toward the foot of the bed to see Haylie like I did every morning. She gave me kisses and pawed my hands like she always did, and it was around that time I noticed it. The weird green boogers in her nose. Did dogs get green boogers? I mean, I guess dogs get green boogers. *Apparently* dogs get green boogers.

She sounded a little congested when she breathed and just gave off the vibe that she didn't feel awesome that day. We went about our morning routine; coffee, treats, meditation, reading, writing (yes, it's a long routine), and once I was caffeinated and functioning I did my best to clean out her nose with a washcloth and some warm water. It didn't seem to help much, but I thought it brought her some kind of minor relief.

Throughout the day Haylie seemed to be more tired and lethargic than usual, not getting up to come visit me while I worked, not getting up when she heard food wrappers in the kitchen. Not eating much, but to be fair, her eating still hadn't normalized since she finished chemo a month and a half before. By the time four o'clock in the afternoon rolled around, I was dialing her vet in tears because she was acting so out of character, had barely gotten out of bed all day, and just was generally seeming not at all okay. With the agreement that if things changed during the night I would take her to the emergency vet, we scheduled an appointment for her first thing the next morning. One of us didn't sleep that night.

At her morning appointment, it was determined between the green boogers and congestion and lethargy that she likely had an upper respiratory infection. Haylie was put on two weeks of antibiotics and I was instructed to monitor her and let her rest. While I was fascinated by the amount of green boogers that could come out of one dog's nose, I was also relieved that this was something so relatively minor that could be treated easily.

The next morning around ten o'clock, I noticed Haylie wouldn't even drink water. She tried to, she'd put her mouth down in the bowl, but she'd immediately lift her head back up like she couldn't do it. Again, I called the vet, wondering if she had drainage from her nose going down her throat and it was causing her to have a sore throat. The on-call vet said it was possible and prescribed a nose drop that would help break up the green boogery mess sooner so that hopefully she could move through this more quickly.

As the day wore on, she began sounding more and more congested and hoarse. She was awake more than she had been in a couple days, but only because she was panting hard with this raspy sound that didn't so much sound like an upper respiratory infection as a pig with a heavy cigarette addiction. When she was resting, it wasn't so bad. But when she was away, it sounded like the pig had been smoking for at least 30 years, maybe longer.

I monitored her for the rest of the day and once I finished my work day my dad came over to see her himself, since I was on the fence about taking her to the emergency hospital. She didn't have this raspy, scratchy breathing thing going on when she saw her doctor a day or two before, so this was a new development, and one I wasn't super comfortable with. She seemed to be straining to breathe altogether.

In the spirit of we-don't-know-what-the-hell-is-going-on-and-we're-not-doctors, we decided to take Haylie to the emergency vet. They took her to the back within a few minutes of examining her since she was in "respiratory distress." We waited.

They said her throat was very swollen, that she was breathing through a space the size of a tiny straw. We waited.

They said they gave her a steroid injection to hopefully bring the swelling down. We waited.

They said the swelling could be due to a number of things, but it was likely her lymphoma was back, in the lymph nodes in her neck, causing the inflammation. They wanted to do further testing and gather further information and would have her for several hours. We went home. And waited.

It was nine o'clock at night by the time we got home, and I changed into my pajamas as if everything was normal and got in bed to read, only to find I had no attention span and only a laser focus on the fact that Haylie wasn't at the foot of my bed like she had been nearly every night for the last 13 years. I cried. I stopped. I checked to see if my phone still worked. I cried some more. Eventually I dozed off with all the lights on, to be woken up by a phone call around midnight.

This is the time when I tell you I didn't realize there would be parts of this book that would be so difficult to write. There are tears on my keyboard as I type the words that came out of the phone, *"She's not in good shape. The steroid is not helping with the swelling. I've intubated her because she's not breathing well on her own. And I need permission to perform a tracheotomy if she doesn't extubate well or continue breathing on her own afterward. It's an invasive procedure, she's 13 years old, this is where we talk about quality of life."*

In shock, but without hesitation, I told the doctor to do what she had to do. Not only could I not lose Haylie, but she had just finished chemotherapy. She had *just* beat cancer. She had so much life left in her to live.

The next day, having extubated well and made it through the night with no more drama, a CT scan revealed that it didn't, in fact, look like her cancer was back, it looked like there was a foreign object in her throat, dug into the tissues, which caused the swelling. She would need it surgically removed. In the meantime, the steroid had finally worked its way through the tremendous amount of swelling in her throat and begun decreasing it. She woke up from the sedation for CT able to breathe close to normally on her own. Her doctor said if I felt comfortable, and would bring her back if things started to flare up again, I could take her home for the night while we regrouped and got surgery scheduled.

I got her home and didn't leave her side, but I started to notice something else different about her. As her excitement to be home and back with me wore off, she could no longer get the back of her body, her back legs, up by herself. *She could no longer stand up by herself.*

The doctor said several episodes of sedation would likely cause this and that as the sedation fully wears off, I should see improvement. But I didn't. She peed after lying down for a while because she could no longer get up on her own and go to the door to tell me she needed to go outside. Soon she was wearing diapers day and night. I lifted her off the bed in the morning. She'd walk around a little and then lay down. Every couple of hours, she'd sit up and I'd lift her butt up for her so she could walk around again and stretch out her muscles, use her legs. Then she'd lay back down and we'd repeat this all day long. I took her diaper off one afternoon and she went out in the yard to go potty. I went inside to answer a phone call and came back out to find her underneath the deck, where she had sat down and couldn't get back up to come to me when I called her. There was such fear in her eyes, my heart shattered into a million pieces when I found her. I crawled under the deck, scratching myself up to help her stand and get her back inside. Once we were up, her back legs gave out on the stairs into the apartment and she fell onto her butt looking confused and terrified and helpless all at once. The million pieces of my heart shattered into a million more.

In the end, by some miracle, the doctors determined they truly didn't know for certain *why* her throat swelled up but the swelling never came back so she got to ditch the surgery to avoid an invasive procedure for no apparent reason. After a set of x-rays on her hips revealed arthritis, an anti-inflammatory + pain med got her back on her feet and bouncing around like a puppy again.

But I spent several weeks changing her diapers, helping her up and down the stairs, lifting up her butt for her so she could stand, and waking up in the middle of the night just to lay with her and listen to her breathe. This creature that I had always gone to for comfort, that had saved my life, that had gently but surely kept me going year after year, needed me to help keep her going, in a very literal sense. It took everything in me and brought out strength I didn't know I had, and at times I just laid with her and cried over how painful the experience of watching her diminish was. People do it with parents every single day, and I look up to them, because those few weeks destroyed me. The world around me stopped and nothing mattered but taking care of her. And I know there will come a day when I will face this again with her.

And I will be honored to be the one to change her diapers all the way to the end.

10 Reasons Dogs Are the Absolute Best

"Life is a series of dogs." G. Carlin

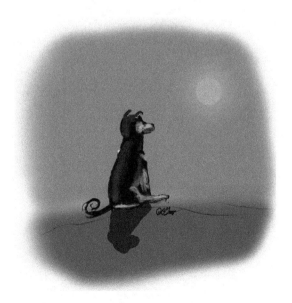

10 Reasons Dogs Are the Absolute Best

've been through many with my family. There was Bear, the white German Shepherd, who was my protector when I was born. Then Prancer, the black German Shepherd, who pranced instead of walked. There was Gretta, the three-legged German Shepherd, Hal, the Rottweiler, whom I ran away with at about 16 or 17 years old, and Button, the little blonde Border Collie mix. Now there's Socks, the black we're-not-quite-sure mix with white socks on his feet, and Louie, the handsome but slightly goofy German Shepherd with traditional markings. My sister has been through two dogs of her own in the time I've had Haylie and is now raising her third, a beautiful, all black, timid, sweet girl named Guinness (yes, after the darkest of dark beers). My other sister has two, Desi the Schnauzer and Lucy the Schnorkie, both loves of her life in tiny, furry packages.

There's been beach vacations with them and bath time and late nights and early mornings. Emergencies (more than we can count) and holidays and food stolen off the counters and off of plates and off of picnic tables and off of anything else you can think of (mostly Haylie). There's been dogs off on adventures by themselves (aka lost) and late night searches and bickering between them and unique personalities belonging to each of them.

And of course, there's been goodbyes. Lots of goodbyes. Heart-wrenching, soul-crushing goodbyes. I don't remember saying goodbye to Bear because I was too little, so my first memorable goodbye was Prancer, who we got when I was around two and put down when I was 16. I just remember having such a clear realization that I had never felt so much pain in my life, visceral, aching pain, emotional and physical. My heart hurt for weeks.

For Mother's Day this year, I wrote and published an article called *My Child Has Paws, and Here's Why She Still Counts on Mother's Day.* I shared it to Facebook and a friend commented with one of the most beautiful perspectives I've ever heard: that we have the privilege of seeing this big love between dog and human through, from beginning to end.

I've spent a lot of time thinking about this perspective, and wrapping my head around it, and trying to adopt it. The truth is, I still don't know how I'll make it through losing Haylie when the time comes. People continue telling me you just somehow get through it, and I'm choosing to believe them, because I have no faith in my own ability to live in a world without her when she's the reason I stayed in this world so many times. But when I think of it in terms of myself and Haylie showing each other love full circle, from beginning to end, it comforts my heart in the strangest, most welcome way. Because it makes me realize I've given her something invaluable, the biggest love I have, and if I can give her even half of what she's given me in her time with me on this earth, I will be honored.

There's no magic fairy dust or perfect words to make the loss of a dog more bearable or easier or less painful. But to know you're honoring their love by seeing them through to the end, is a gift we can give them after they've given us so much in their lifetimes. As my favorite dog quote at the beginning of this book says, they give us their all; giving them love full circle is a beautiful, transparent way we can give back.

CH. 10 They love *love*

"It's just the most amazing thing to love a dog, isn't it? It makes our relationships with people seem as boring as a bowl of oatmeal." J. Grogan

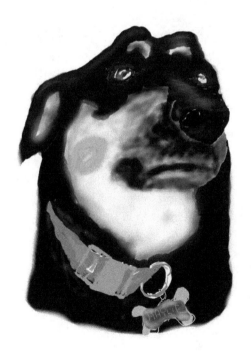

10 Reasons Dogs Are the Absolute Best

I've heard the saying *'dogs are the only creatures on earth that love others more than they love themselves.'*

Let's give them a run for their hypothetical money and show them our love: use the next few pages to write your dog or dogs a love letter. Forget my reasons that you've just read; tell them the reasons *you* think they're the absolute best. Tell them about the gifts they've given you. Tell them about your favorite times with them, what you love the most about them, and how they've changed your life.

Write to them as if they're a person and understand every word, because I believe when you read it to them, *they will.*

Keep the letter (whether you write it in this book or in a separate journal or notebook pages) in a place you can revisit it once in a while, reminding you of the preciousness and bigness of this love between you. Maybe even create a tradition out of it and write *all* of your dogs a love letter when they enter your life and when they leave your life. At the end of your life, you'll have a box of letters that prove beyond a shadow of a doubt that you experienced one of the most pure, non-judgmental, unconditional loves to exist - multiplied by however many dogs you've loved in your lifetime.

Now *that* is a beautiful life.

10 Reasons Dogs Are the Absolute Best

_____

_____

_____

_____

_____

_____

_____

_____

_____

_____

_____

_____

_____

_____

_____

10 Reasons Dogs Are the Absolute Best

_____

_____

_____

_____

_____

_____

_____

_____

_____

_____

_____

_____

_____

_____

10 Reasons Dogs Are the Absolute Best

About Dublin's Dream Dog Rescue

"Until they all find a home."

25% of all proceeds for the book you hold in your hands go to non-profit organization Dublin's Dream Dog Rescue.

I was raised with rescue dogs. I've never met a rescue dog I didn't like. So when it came time to decide where to donate a portion of profits for this book, there was only one option: a dog rescue!

Unfortunately, it wasn't that easy.

I Googled dog rescues and found pages upon pages of deserving ones, some more popular with huge followings and YouTube Channels and others smaller and lesser known. But none tugged at my heart the way Dublin's Dream did when I first came across them.

I'd had professional photos taken with Haylie the month I began writing this book and became friends with my photographer on Facebook (because who doesn't love someone who spends all day photographing dogs?). I found Dublin's Dream on her page and instantly felt drawn to the rescue organization and the beautiful faces that lined their feed, puppies and adults alike.

Dublin's Dream is located in Reno, Nevada, and serves the Northern Nevada and California areas. Named after a very special Red Rhodesian Ridgeback mix, Dublin's dream is for all dogs to get their happily-ever-after.

You can learn more about Dublin's Dream Dog Rescue at Facebook.com/dublinsdreamrescue

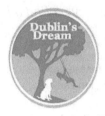

About the Author

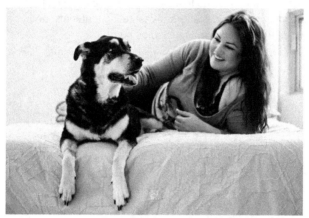

Photo by Christy Arias

Amanda Gist is a first-time author, passionate storyteller, thunderstorm lover, and mac and cheese aficionado.

She writes and speaks on a wide range of topics, from the rescue dog that saved her to difficult conversations about mental health and eating disorders. Her passion is personal growth topics like self-compassion, feeding your soul, finding your truth, and learning to get back up after a dream has been shattered.

What she's good at: being a dog mom, making animals out of Play-Doh, listening, cooking steak, bringing love to email inboxes *(www.amandagist.com)*, and setting monthly intentions with each new moon.

What she's working on: working less and living more, yoga, cooking salmon, regularly watering her plants, and actually reading her giant list of books to read.

Amanda is also the owner of *Soulful Creative Studios,* a copywriting studio specializing in writing for heart-centered and spiritual entrepreneurs and brands. She works with clients to bring a voice to all kinds of projects, from blogs to websites, email newsletters to marketing materials, and more. *(www.soulfulcreativestudios.com)*

Acknowledgements

Writing my first book has been an effort contributed to by many. I have so many people to thank for moral support, hands-on help, and listening to me talk endlessly about writing along the way.

To Dad, thank you for the beautiful illustrations (all 482,609 of them), the book talks along the way, for asking me how it was going, for helping me from beginning to end, and for being an inspiration to achieve my goals. I did it!!

To Mom, you listened to me talk about this book for six weeks straight. Your patience is unmatched. Thank you for always pushing me to reach for the stars.

To Meg, you were the very first to read the manuscript, the moment I asked you to. Thank you for always stepping up to help me when I need you and for being there. You're the best sweater a girl could ask for.

To Lyndsey, your dream was right – I wrote a book. Maybe not the one we both thought, but hopefully it is the first of many.

To Aunt Sandy, I DID SOMETHING I'M PROUD OF!

To Lindsey and Alex, thank you for fully facilitating the first dream come true for me in many, many years. You believed in me when I questioned myself, my topic, my abilities, my hair, my face, everything (which was immediately) and provided dog pics when I needed them the most. I can never thank you enough.

To Jillian, I hope you read this book to Coco and I hope she loves it. You've been a welcome surprise in my life since the day you made that donation, and your support is unwavering. Don't forget our pool house deal.

To Lela, I don't think we talked about this book once, but your name in Skype every day lit up long hours this summer. Thank you. <3

To Celia and Brenda, thank you for being a part of my healing and helping me reach a point in my life where I can, like, write. a. book. There were many times I never thought being a productive human being would be possible for me. You both helped me get there.

To Christy and Furever, thank you for the experience of a lifetime with my little one. I will forever love that we got some of my favorite shots because of Haylie's stubbornness.

To Dr. Emina, you told me my creativity would come back, over and over. And I didn't believe you, over and over. I'm so happy I was wrong and you were right. Thank you.

To Michelle, thank you for always making sure I have the magic stuff that helps me live. And for the Big Dog stories and pictures. They have brightened my life.

Last but not least, to Haylie Denae, thank you for the love, inspiration, and for saving me baby girl. You will always, always have my heart.

Closing Thoughts

"Dogs' lives are too short. Their only fault, really." A. Turnbull

In closing, maybe this book has made you smile. Maybe it's made you cry. Maybe it's made you look at your dog a little differently. My hope is that it's given you a reminder of all the ways they show up in our lives while we're busy living them. A reminder of all of your own stories, the ones that make up the beautiful thread of life you've lived with your own dog or dogs.

The big love between human and dog is so uncomplicated, so untethered, so pure, it can withstand the deepest of valleys and the highest of peaks. They don't bail when things get hard, they get closer to us. They don't judge us at our worst, they love us at our worst. They owe us nothing, yet they give us everything.

And when the sun sets on their final day, when our eyes are filled with tears and our hearts are filled with aching, visceral pain and sorrow, I hope we can all remember our full circle love. The silent promise that we made to them when we brought them home, to root them into our hearts forever and see them through to the end.

Both times I almost lost Haylie, when she was diagnosed with b-cell lymphoma and given a month to live without chemo, and when her throat closed up nine months later, one of the hardest questions I needed an answer to was this: *How will I ever get another dog? How will I ever replace her?*

I find comfort in my dad's words, *"You never replace them, you love them all differently."*

They Will Not Go Quietly

They will not go quietly,
the pets who've shared our lives.
In subtle ways they let us know
their spirit still survives.
Old habits still can make us think
we hear them at the door
Or step back when we drop
a tasty morsel on the floor.
Our feet still go around the place
the food dish used to be.
And, sometimes, coming home at night,
we miss them terribly.
And although time may bring new friends
and a new food dish to fill,
That one place in our hearts belongs to them...
and always will.

- Unknown

10 Reasons Dogs Are the Absolute Best

CPSIA information can be obtained
at www.ICGtesting.com
Printed in the USA
LVHW080806310720
661951LV00006B/98